BREATHE

Restoring Natural Breathing According to Your Body's Design and Improve Physical, Mental, and Emotional Health

By Joey Lott

www.joeylott.com

Publishing services provided by **Archangel Ink**

ISBN: 151866587X
ISBN-13: 978-1518665875

Table of Contents

4

The Purpose of this Book

Breathing. Who would have thought that so much could be said about something so natural and so seemingly simple? Why on earth would anyone need or want to learn how to breathe? Shouldn't we breathe correctly without instruction? And what's the big deal if we don't? It can't matter all that much, can it? Isn't it just a matter of breathing in and out?

For better or worse (and for the most part, it's been for the worse) I have taken an interest in breathing for a little over 15 years. And in that time, I've learned and tried some stupid and downright dangerous breathing practices. I know I'm not the only one. Plus, in the name of improving my health, I tried all kinds of practices that, if done correctly, *could* have been beneficial. However, since the level of instruction was consistently poor or incomplete, I never learned to do them correctly. Instead, I compounded my problems by misusing respiratory muscles and over-breathing.

Our anatomy and biology dictate that there is a *normal* way to breathe. Other ways of breathing are possible. However, they will produce suboptimal results. When done incorrectly, the act of breathing can actually produce health problems.

When I say that there is a normal way to breathe, I am not suggesting that it is universally correct in all situations. Rather, human anatomy and biology dictate that when at rest – and barring unusual circumstances – there is one optimal way to breathe. Modifications of that pattern may be appropriate under other circumstances, of course. For example, during high levels of physical exertion, the pattern of breathing will be different than when at rest. But in most cases, the pattern isn't dramatically different. This book will explore normal breathing in hopes that it may be helpful to you.

I now cringe a little when I see how many times poor breathing advice or instruction is doled out. This ranges from yoga classes to self-help courses to advice from psychologists to friends advising friends to "take a deep breath."

I cringe because nine times out of 10 it seems to me that the advice or instruction prompts the recipients to *over* breathe. Breathing too much can have catastrophic health effects when practiced for long periods of time. The scientific term for over-breathing is *hyperventilation*. We'll be taking a look at hyperventilation in a lot more detail throughout the book, and by the end, you will understand why it is a problem and how to take some simple, safe, and practical steps to restore normal breathing patterns.

It took the better part of 15 years before I finally took the time to learn just a little bit about the anatomy and the biology of breathing. And when I did, my view of breathing changed. No longer did dramatic and extreme breathing practices appeal to me. No longer did I follow the instruction to breathe deeply by taking a bigger breath. And I began to see the association between emotional and psychological symptoms and breathing patterns.

In this book, I hope to share with you what I have learned. I don't profess to be the world's leading authority on the subject of breathing. But I can tell you that everything I share in this book is safe, gentle, and founded upon an understanding of how human respiration works. Not all books about breathing can make that claim. In fact, from my experience, far too many should come with a warning that following the advice given in the book is likely to lead to predictable symptoms of hyperventilation.

Other breathing philosophies may offer a lot of theories about how practices will increase Qi or Prana or cleanse you of toxins. I don't dismiss the possibility of Qi or Prana. But many of the exercises that some so-called experts give for raising Qi or Prana lead to hyperventilation, not an increase in energy, at least not in the long term. Also, many of those systems have been traditionally taught in person by genuine masters who have perfected some technique over a lifetime. Outside of that context, many extreme breathing practices have the potential to be dangerous.

The first thing that I cover in this book is how breathing actually works. I believe this information can offer important insights that will enable you to understand why many breathing practices are harmful, and why restoring normal, healthy breathing is beneficial.

In these initial discussions of anatomy and biology, I use a lot of scientific terms. I do my best to break it down into a simple presentation. At the same time, I know that not everyone enjoyed biology classes in school (I know I didn't). So if you find that material too dry, feel free to skip ahead to the practical sections.

The Anatomy of Breath

For most of us, when we think of breathing, we think first of the lungs. The lungs certainly play a vital role in respiration. However, contrary to popular belief, the lungs play a passive, not an active role in the mechanics of breathing. I frequently hear or read about practices or devices which claim they will "strengthen the lungs." This is a false and misleading claim because the lungs are not muscles.

The lungs are similar to balloons, in many respects. In fact, I have seen a demonstration in which the lungs of a sheep were blown up just like balloons. I am most certainly not suggesting that it is advisable to hyperinflate the lungs, because that can damage delicate tissues in these organs. However, the lungs have a natural elasticity that plays an important role in normal, healthy breathing. Yet on their own, they are incapable of drawing a breath. They rely upon respiratory muscles to do that work.

While there are many muscles that can and do play a role in respiration, they can roughly be grouped into principal respiratory and accessory respiratory muscles. And what many of us will find is that we have relied too much upon accessory respiratory muscles. This can cause some problems.

First, let's look at some of the accessory respiratory muscles. It is possible to breathe using muscles in the neck (sternocleidomastoid muscles), the upper back and chest (internal and external intercostal muscles), and the abdomen. The sternocleidomastoid and external intercostal muscles can all be used to increase the volume of an inhalation, while the abdominal muscles and the internal intercostal muscles can be used to cause a forced exhalation.

Relying heavily on auxiliary respiratory muscles is a mistake for several reasons. Firstly, this exhausts and stresses these muscles, which produces stress, inflammation, and other problems in the body. Secondly, using auxiliary respiratory muscles as your main mode of breathing increases the likelihood of hyperventilation.

The principal respiratory muscle is the thoracic diaphragm. Technically, the external intercostal muscles are sometimes considered to be principal *and* accessory respiratory muscles. However, my own experience is that they are not needed for principal respiration when at rest, and there is no benefit in stressing them unnecessarily. For that reason, I don't consider them to be principal respiratory muscles for the purposes of this book.

The thoracic diaphragm, which I will simply refer to as the diaphragm from now on, is a dome-shaped muscle that attaches at the base of the ribcage. This muscle separates the thoracic cavity (the ribcage) from the abdomen. When the diaphragm contracts, it flattens out into something that more closely resembles a pancake than a dome or bell. This action compresses the abdomen while expanding the thoracic cavity. The change in pressure caused by the increase in thoracic volume has the effect of drawing air into the lungs.

At this point, it is worth clarifying an important point about the structure and function of muscles. Muscles are only capable of working actively in one direction. They contract, or shorten, which draws the ends of the muscles together. For example, the bicep muscles contract and cause the arm to hinge closed at the elbow. A muscle cannot exert force in two directions. Therefore, apart from contracting, the only other thing that a muscle can do is relax or lengthen passively. In other words, the bicep muscles cannot force an arm to hinge open. That action occurs either passively by means of gravity or another external force or by the force of an opposing muscle, such as the tricep muscles.

The diaphragm, like other muscles, moves in one direction by contracting. Otherwise, it can only move passively. When the diaphragm releases, it returns to its neutral position, forming a dome shape. This occurs when the muscle is relaxed.

Therefore, the action of the diaphragm on exhalation is to relax and allow the muscle fibers to lengthen. That means that normal, restful exhalations require absolutely no muscular effort. The air is expelled naturally from a combination of the elastic quality of the lungs and the diaphragm returning to its neutral position and reducing the volume of the thoracic cavity.

Using a process called spirometry (literally the measurement of breath), researchers measure the volumes of air that enter and exit the lungs during respiration. During quiet respiration, this is called tidal volume. On average, in healthy adults the tidal volume is around 12 percent of lung capacity. That means a relatively small amount of air moves in and out of the lungs with each breath, when breathing normally. This is significant because although it is possible to forcefully increase the amount of air that moves in and out with each breath, the effects are not generally desirable. We will look at this in more detail in the following sections.

The Biology of Breath

Physiological respiration refers to the exchange of gasses through the act of breathing. When you inhale, this draws air into your lungs. Within the lungs are millions of tiny structures called alveoli, and these structures transfer gasses – oxygen and carbon dioxide – between the lungs and the blood.

Perhaps the most common explanation of respiration is that it involves the exchange of oxygen into the blood and carbon dioxide out of the blood. This is accurate, but taken alone it is imprecise and misleading. Many people misunderstand this to mean that respiration necessarily entails the exhalation of large amounts of carbon dioxide. In fact, many people refer to carbon dioxide as a "waste product."

But the actual story is different. Humans require both oxygen *and* carbon dioxide. Viewing carbon dioxide as a waste product is overly simplistic. Although we typically exhale more carbon dioxide than we inhale, it is *not* true that we exhale pure carbon dioxide, as is commonly misunderstood. If that was the case, then artificial respiration would not work. Air on earth at sea level contains about 21 percent oxygen and 0.04 percent carbon dioxide, whereas the average air exhaled by humans contains 14 percent oxygen and 5 percent carbon dioxide. In both cases, the vast majority of air is composed of nitrogen.

When you consider the implications of these numbers, along with the tidal volume to total lung capacity ratio, you will soon realize that the human body purposefully increases the carbon dioxide concentration of the air in the lungs. So far from being purely a waste product, carbon dioxide is an essential component of the contents of the lungs.

The body strongly prefers to maintain the 5 percent carbon dioxide content of the lungs; so much so that if the concentration drops significantly, then the lungs will draw more carbon dioxide from the blood. When this process occurs, the blood pH increases, meaning it becomes more alkaline. The increase in pH is due to the fact that carbon dioxide, which is acidic, is being removed from the blood, leaving an imbalance in favor of alkaline substances such as bicarbonate. When the blood becomes overly alkaline due to problems with respiration, it is called respiratory alkalosis. We'll cover this in more detail in the Hyperventilation section, but know that it's not a good thing.

Hyperventilation

Hyperventilation, literally over-breathing, refers to any breathing in excess of metabolic demands. This can occur either by breathing excessively rapidly, or by breathing an excessive volume of air. Breathing in excess of metabolic demands will dilute the carbon dioxide concentration in the lungs. The result is that the lungs will begin to compensate by drawing carbon dioxide from the blood, creating an imbalance.

In a healthy person, the rate and volume of breathing is dictated by the need to expel excess carbon dioxide. This occurs when the body detects that carbon dioxide levels in the lungs have exceeded the desired concentration. This will trigger an inhalation followed by a relaxed, passive exhalation when at rest.

The amount of carbon dioxide in the lungs is determined in part by breathing rate and volume, and in part by the amount of carbon dioxide produced through cellular respiration (i.e. metabolism). Various circumstances such as physical exertion can temporarily increase metabolic rate. Even eating will create a mild increase in metabolic rate. The result is that breathing will naturally increase to compensate for the increased carbon dioxide production.

If carbon dioxide production increases beyond the body's ability to maintain the ideal carbon dioxide concentrations, then the body may compensate through forceful breathing with both exaggerated inhalations and forced exhalations. Typically, this is a good indicator that one should reduce exertion levels to avoid strain, stress, and the possibility of hyperventilation due to lack of control over exaggerated breathing movements.

There are situations in which people may hyperventilate either acutely or chronically. Acute hyperventilation often occurs under stress, and hyperventilation is associated with anxiety and panic episodes. Chronic hyperventilation occurs when a person forms the habit of over-breathing. This is often the result of breathing before the onset of air hunger (i.e. rapid breathing) and/or exceeding normal tidal volume through the overuse of accessory respiratory muscles.

When a person hyperventilates chronically, this makes it extremely easy to suffer an acute hyperventilation episode, which is often interpreted as extreme anxiety or panic. Both chronic and acute hyperventilation can produce symptoms. And because chronic hyperventilation can be relatively subtle, it is often difficult to detect, except when one becomes educated and familiar with the patterns and sensations of normal breathing.

As mentioned in the previous section, hyperventilation can produce alkalosis, which means that the pH of the blood increases beyond the normal range. The blood contains carbon dioxide (CO_2, which is acidic) and bicarbonate (HCO_3, which is alkaline). When the lungs draw carbon dioxide from the blood to maintain the concentrations in the lungs, this produces an alkaline state, because the ratio of bicarbonate to carbon dioxide increases. In the short term, the body compensates for this imbalance by converting bicarbonate to carbon dioxide and water by combining it with free hydrogen ions to form carbonic acid (H_2CO_3), which is then processed by an enzyme to produce carbon dioxide (CO_2) and water (H_2O).

Since respiratory alkalosis forces the body to compensate for the excess alkalinity, several undesirable effects ensue. For one thing, it causes something called the Bohr effect, which causes hemoglobin to bind more tightly with oxygen. The result is that oxygen levels in the tissues decrease. Generally speaking, this is not desirable.

The process of converting bicarbonate to carbon dioxide results in a decrease of free hydrogen atoms in the blood. Both hydrogen ions and calcium ions can bind with albumin. When the number of free hydrogen ions reduces, more calcium binds to albumin. Since the free calcium ions are the form of biologically active calcium in the blood, the result is low levels of usable calcium, a condition known as hypocalcemia.

Alkalosis can initiate an increase in glycosis, which is a process that requires a large amount of phosphate. The result is that phosphate is removed from the blood to feed this process. The drop in phosphate in the blood is called hypophosphatemia.

In the long term, in cases of chronic hyperventilation, the body will begin to compensate by excreting bicarbonate through the kidneys. The result may be further electrolyte depletion as well as changes to kidney function that provide short-term survival, but reduce efficiency.

Because the effects of hyperventilation are so extensive, the symptoms can be quite varied. In the acute stages the most common effects are lightheadedness, dizziness, faintness, and palpitations. However, the symptoms can also include cold hands and feet, confusion, blurred vision, depersonalization, chest pain, breathlessness, increased urination, parasthesia, "pins and needles," and tetany (involuntary muscular contractions).

Hyperventilation, whether acute or chronic, produces compensatory measures that allow one to survive. However, that does not mean that it is a desirable state. All evidence shows that the ideal condition is one where breathing perfectly matches metabolic needs. In the next section, we'll look at what normal breathing is.

Normal Breathing

As I suggested in the previous section, normal, healthy breathing is efficient breathing. The most efficient breathing is that which perfectly matches the metabolic needs at the moment.

Breathing, also known as the mechanical portion of respiration, serves several purposes, but perhaps the two most important are fueling cellular respiration with the input of oxygen and removing excess carbon dioxide build-up. In other words, the rate at which you breathe should ideally be dictated by the need for oxygen and the need to remove excess carbon dioxide. In practice, since there is usually an abundance of oxygen (even expelled air is still relatively oxygen-rich), the body relies almost exclusively on carbon dioxide levels to regulate the breath.

The implication of a carbon dioxide-regulated breath is that the normal pattern of healthy breathing is one in which the onset of mild air hunger initiates the next inhalation. That means that in normal breathing at rest, there will be a natural pause at the bottom of the exhalation, and only when air hunger arises will the next inhalation occur. The duration of the pause can range anywhere from a second to 10 seconds or more. Of course, you should not attempt to force this pause. (There are some practices that can be done safely that do incorporate a breath hold between the exhalation and the inhalation. However, for reasons that I will provide later, I don't recommend this as a practice until you have mastered the basics and become very familiar with the patterns and sensations of healthy, normal breathing.)

You will also recall from the discussion of breathing anatomy that when one uses the diaphragm correctly, the inhalation will be active and the exhalation will be passive. That is because the diaphragm flattens when it contracts, drawing air into the lungs, while the exhalation phase is produced by the passive return of the diaphragm to its relaxed dome shape combined with the natural elasticity of the lungs. So when you exhale normally, you should experience a complete relaxation of all respiratory muscles. Normal exhalations are *not* forced.

The combination of a passive exhalation and a relatively infrequent need for air means that in normal breathing, the exhalations are much slower than the inhalations.

The final component of normal breathing is that it occurs through the nose as opposed to the mouth. Nasal breathing warms, filters, and moistens the incoming air, making it easier for the body to assimilate. When breathing through the mouth, it is possible that incoming air will be too cool or too dry for the body to utilize.

Mouth breathing increases the likelihood of hyperventilation. While it is possible to breathe normal volumes and at normal rates through the mouth, breathing through the nose makes it easier to regulate volume and rate.

Nasal breathing produces nitric oxide in the sinuses. Mouth breathing does not. Nitric oxide plays an important role in breathing. It is antibacterial, which means that nasal breathing filters incoming air not only mechanically through nose hairs, but also chemically with nitric oxide. And nitric oxide is a vasodilator (a relaxant of blood vessels) and a bronchodilator (a relaxant of the bronchioles, which are the conduits to the alveoli), which means that it can help produce more efficient respiration by making it easier for the air to reach the alveoli.

And lastly, normal breathing is regular and rhythmic. Of course, changes in metabolic demands will produce expected changes in breathing. For example, you might expect that your breathing will change in a predictable way when you walk versus when you are at rest. However, at every point your breathing should be complete and rhythmic, even if that rhythm changes. Erratic breathing is indicative of either health problems or poor habits. Each complete inhalation should be followed by a complete exhalation. That is not to say that either inhalation or exhalation should be forced. However, unhealthy, erratic breathing may involve a series of partial inhalations interspersed with partial exhalations, creating an a-rhythmic, chaotic breathing pattern.

In summary, normal resting breathing has the following characteristics:

- The inhalation is through the nose. Exhalation is typically through the nose as well, though the evidence is not as strong as to suggest that the benefits of exhalation through the nose are as great as for inhalation through the nose.
- Inhalations use the diaphragm as the principal respiratory muscle.
- Exhalations are longer than inhalations.
- Exhalations are relaxed and passive.
- At the end of each exhalation, there is a pause until air hunger prompts the next inhalation.
- Breathing is regular and rhythmic.

Diagnosing Breathing Health

Now that you've had a chance to learn about both normal and abnormal breathing, as well as some of the drawbacks of abnormal breathing, you may want to determine the quality of your own breathing at rest. This will give you a sense of what your breathing habits are, and what, if anything, you might want to improve.

The first and most obvious thing you can check is whether you are breathing through your nose or your mouth. Some people are chronic mouth breathers, breathing through the mouth even when at rest. Other people breathe through the mouth only during exertion, such as when walking. And still other people breathe through the mouth while sleeping. None of these patterns are optimal or part of a normal breathing pattern. So if you find that you breathe through your mouth, make an effort to keep it closed and breathe through the nose instead. If necessary, reduce the exertion by slowing your pace, reducing the load, or taking breaks as necessary.

Forming a habit of nasal breathing while asleep can be a bit more challenging. Some people find that a few pieces of strategically placed medical tape help to gently "remind" the mouth to stay shut without mechanically preventing air from getting in and out of the mouth, if necessary. Other people find that a chin strap designed for use with a Continuous Positive Airways Pressure (CPAP) machine works to keep the mouth shut well enough.

The next easiest thing to diagnose is the muscles you are using to breathe. The simple test is to place one hand on your abdomen and one hand on your chest. Breathe as you usually do, and notice the movement of the two hands. Ideally, only your abdomen will move while your chest will remain mostly motionless.

In regard to muscles used for breathing, there are a handful of scenarios that can present themselves. Again, the ideal is when the abdomen moves while the chest is relatively still. The abdomen should move down and out slightly on inhalation, and it should return to a neutral position on exhalation. However, other dysfunctional patterns can and do often occur. One such pattern is for both the abdomen and the chest to expand on inhalation. While a small expansion in the chest is not normally problematic, an exaggerated expansion indicates overuse of the intercostal muscles and hyperventilation.

Another common dysfunctional pattern is one in which the chest moves while the abdomen is still or perhaps even worse, the abdomen may draw in on the inhalation in a pattern known as reverse breathing. This indicates a gross misuse of respiratory muscles. In this scenario, the person is likely to feel short of breath, anxious, fatigued, and possibly feel tightness in the chest.

One more common pattern involves a forced exhalation. This pattern may involve a drawing in of the abdomen on exhalation, a tightening of the chest on exhalation, or both. This pattern of breathing is likely to lead to fatigue and tightness. It also is very likely to lead to hyperventilation.

Another useful diagnostic is to count the number of seconds of your usual inhalation and exhalation. In normal breathing, the inhalation will be relatively short – likely just a few seconds – and the exhalation will be relatively longer. If your exhalations are not notably longer than your inhalations, then this is likely an indicator of a less than optimal breathing pattern.

You can also count the number of breaths per minute to get an idea of the rate at which you breathe. The definitions of healthy respiration rates vary greatly, depending on who you ask. Johns Hopkins Medical School suggests that anywhere from 12 to 16 breaths per minute is normal and healthy. Other medical organizations suggest that anywhere from 10 to 20 breaths per minute is normal. On the other hand, other traditions of breathing instruction suggest much lower ranges from 5 to 10 breaths per minute.

I don't believe that these ranges are very helpful, except for on the high end. If you are breathing more than 20 times per minute at rest, then this is a fairly strong indicator of hyperventilation. Otherwise, I believe that tuning into the cues of genuine air hunger and letting that prompt the inhalation, instead of breathing merely out of habit, is the best course of action.

With that said, in my own experience, I have found that relaxed, conscious, optimal breathing patterns *tend* to involve low respiratory rates on the scale of 5 to 10 breaths per minute. I don't believe that the goal should be to artificially lower the respiratory rate simply because it is thought to be "better" in some way. Rather, the goal should be to relax and tune in to the natural cues that prompt normal breathing. For most of us, that will naturally result in a more relaxed, slower respiratory rate than we have probably become accustomed to through habit.

Developing Diaphragmatic Breathing

For most of us, diaphragmatic breathing would appear to be the natural mode of breathing. And if we manage to remain unscathed and are not otherwise taught to breathe differently, then chances are we will never deviate from the natural mode.

However, a great many of us for one reason or another developed different breathing habits. We lost touch with the natural pattern of diaphragmatic breathing. As a result, most of us are breathing inefficiently, possibly hyperventilating. So the first and most important step in regaining a normal breathing pattern is to reacquaint yourself (or acquaint yourself for the very first time in some cases) with diaphragmatic breathing.

To begin with, one of the simplest ways to familiarize yourself with the sensation of diaphragmatic breathing is to place one hand on the chest and the other on the abdomen. As you breathe, consciously relax the chest.

You want to feel with your hand that the chest is remaining still on inhalation and exhalation. Make sure there is no tension in the chest, either. Do not attempt to force the chest still with muscular tension. Instead, relax it completely and let the breath be gentle and easy.

With each inhalation, feel the hand on your abdomen gently moving outward as the muscles relax. Remember that the diaphragm is between the chest and the abdomen, so the muscles both above and below should remain relaxed. At the top of the inhalation, simply let go of the diaphragmatic contraction and maintain the relaxation in the abdomen. As you do, feel the abdomen gently and slowly return to a neutral position.

As you do this simple exercise, keep the entire body as relaxed as possible. Relax not only the chest and abdomen, but also the jaw, neck, throat, and shoulders. Notice if there is a habit of tensing any of these muscles, particularly at the top of the inhalation. If so, relax even more and reduce the volume of the inhalation ever so slightly.

Eventually, you will become attuned to the subtle movements of respiratory muscles and be able to notice the quality of the breath and whether or not you are breathing diaphragmatically without having to place your hands on your chest and abdomen. This will allow you to be aware of your breath at any time. Since efficient breathing is always a good thing, having awareness of the breath at any time is valuable. You can do this while sitting at a desk, while watching television, while driving, while riding on a train, and even while eating or talking.

Of course we aren't always sedentary, so it is useful to begin to apply this same sort of awareness to the breath while active. Depending on your level of fitness and breathing efficiency, you may notice that breathing diaphragmatically can initially be challenging when walking or doing other types of activity. Don't worry about it. Whenever possible, slow down the pace or reduce the level of exertion, so you can apply the same exercise to your activity. For example, when you are walking, you can place one hand on your chest and another on your abdomen and, just as before, see that your chest is moving very little while your abdomen moves outward gently on the inhalation and returns to neutral on the exhalation. Also, make sure the chest and abdomen remain relaxed throughout.

As I've mentioned, the rate of respiration is likely to increase during activity because the carbon dioxide levels will increase. However, if your goal is to develop healthy diaphragmatic breathing most of the time, including during activity, then you will likely get the best results by reducing the exertion to a manageable level, so that you can breathe with the diaphragm and allow the exhalation to be relaxed. With practice, you will probably find that you will become more capable of greater exertion with relaxed diaphragmatic breathing over time.

Breathe Less

Breathing less (volume) with each breath than you are accustomed to is often a very helpful practice. That is not to say that everyone will benefit from breathing less. However, since a large percentage of people are chronic hyperventilators, the practice of reducing the inhalations slightly can yield benefits.

There are traditions and schools of thought that espouse the benefits of reduced breathing. Two of the most prominent are the Buteyko method and hypoventilation training.

The Buteyko method is a (sometimes) cultish method of breath re-training developed in the last century by a Russian doctor named Konstantin Buteyko. Instructors of the method are sometimes zealous in their approach and can sometimes make large claims such as curing cancer, heart disease and many other conditions through the approach. As you have already hopefully seen in this book, reducing the tendency to hyperventilate can have far reaching health benefits, and so it is at least theoretically possible that reduced breathing training like the Buteyko method could produce a great many improvements, up to and including healing things such as heart disease. However, most of these claims are unverified by Western studies. The few studies that have been conducted show mixed results for asthma, though in most cases, regardless of the measured outcomes, the participants in the studies showed a considerable improvement in their sense of well-being, with a reduction in or elimination of the need for drugs.

The Butyeko method can be very powerful. I have done the exercises, and I have derived benefit from them. And, as far as established methods of breath re-training go, Buteyko is presently the best I know of. My only caution in recommending the method is that individual instructors vary greatly in their approach. Some are very gentle and safe while others use an extreme approach, which could be dangerous. I believe that it is more advisable to practice simple, natural, unforced reduced breathing exercises, as I will outline in this section.

Hypoventilation training is a method of athletic training that is widely used now by professional athletes in order to gain an advantage. Hypoventilation training, or HT, has been used since the 1950s to simulate high-altitude training. One of the most famous early users of the approach was Emil Zatopek, the Czech runner and multi-gold medal Olympic athlete. Since then, HT has been used extensively, and studies show that it gives athletes an improvement in performance of 1 percent to

4 percent in some but not all types of competitive athletic events.

Researchers are still arguing about the theory behind HT as well as the "best" way to perform the exercises. However, one thing shows up consistently in the studies: HT produces an increase in CO_2 concentrations in the lungs, blood, and muscles, and this may be an important factor in the benefits of the approach.

HT involves breath holds that can be potentially detrimental in the long term. As such, HT is not suitable as a practice for most people or as a normal breathing style. However, HT does demonstrate that there are benefits to be had by correcting hyperventilation.

While many breathing philosophies and programs emphasize practice sessions, I believe that the most important factor is how you breathe the majority of the time, not just how you breathe for 20 minutes each day. Of course, setting aside some time to acquaint yourself with a new way of breathing has benefits, and so practice times can be helpful. But my belief is that having awareness of your breath throughout the day is likely to yield the greatest results over time. So I propose modest practice sessions combined with awareness of breath throughout the day. Ideally, there should be little difference between your breathing during and outside of the practice session.

I believe that the very best reduced breathing exercise is one that is relaxed, safe, and gentle. Of course, if your habitual breathing pattern is dysfunctional, there may be an initial adjustment period during which adapting to the new, natural, healthy breathing pattern may be uncomfortable and unfamiliar. However, I don't believe that breath retraining needs to be stressful or extremely uncomfortable. The exercise that I suggest meets these criteria.

In order to perform the reduced breathing exercises, begin with your hands on your chest and abdomen as when learning to breathe diaphragmatically. Relax your neck, shoulders, chest, and abdomen. Allow the effects of gravity to gently relax the entire body so that you can feel the support of the ground beneath you. And turn your attention to your breath. Do not force any changes, but notice the pattern and gently soften and release any holding or tension. Begin to feel your abdomen moving outward slightly on the inhalation, and then gently return to neutral on a relaxed exhalation.

Once you feel comfortable and relaxed in this natural breathing pattern, take note of the amount of air that you draw into the lungs with each inhalation. After several more rounds of breath, reduce the volume of the next inhalation by 10 percent. Continue to breathe in this same manner for several minutes. Maintain a relaxed breathing pattern in which the inhalations are 90 percent of your usual breath.

As you breathe in this manner, you will ideally experience very mild air hunger. This should *not* be stressful. If it is, then you have reduced the volume of the inhalation too much. Your goal is to remain entirely relaxed throughout and to find a reduction in air volume that you can sustain indefinitely.

The mild air hunger that you will likely experience is likely because you are now accumulating a very small increase in carbon dioxide in the lungs. Because your body may be adapted to chronic hyperventilation, it will take a little while before it begins to adjust. However, it will eventually begin to retain bicarbonate and naturally increase the saturation of carbon dioxide in the blood and muscles. When this happens, you will no longer feel any air hunger.

When that happens, you can further reduce the inhalation volume by 10 percent. This should once again create a sensation of very mild air hunger. And again, you should strive to find the reduction in volume that creates a sustainable level of air hunger that is not stressful. This will allow your body to adapt to a slightly higher concentration of carbon dioxide.

Initially, you may find it beneficial to set aside time for a dedicated practice of this exercise. As you become more skilled, you can maintain an awareness of your breath throughout the day and maintain a gently reduced breathing volume.

As with all things, this exercise can be beneficial in moderation, but more is not always better. Breathing is healthy, and there is an ideal breathing volume for each of us at any given moment. If you have been in the habit of hyperventilating, then reducing the volume will produce benefits. But that doesn't mean that it is beneficial to continue to reduce the volume forever. It is possible to make the breath too small. The good news is that biofeedback will serve as your guide in this process. The exercise should never produce stress. At the first signs of stress, listen to your body and ease up a little.

If you experience stress, then eventually your body will force you to breathe more, and that will likely produce a pattern of hyperventilation. So always respect that the exercise should not be stressful. In fact, it should mostly feel good! Although mild air hunger may feel slightly uncomfortable at first, if you do this exercise correctly then the discomfort should yield to relaxation and pleasure, much as gentle stretching may be initially uncomfortable but yield to relaxation. And, like stretching, overdoing it can do harm rather than good. So do reduced breathing exercises slowly, gently, and with kindness to your body. Make this a practice for a lifetime, not something to power through.

Slow Down

Reducing the volume of the breath typically provides the most benefits overall. When the volume is too great, that tends to exacerbate all kinds of problems, including excessive rapidity of the breath. As such, I believe that reducing the volume of the breath is the single best exercise you can do.

Many educators and schools of breathing suggest that slowing the breath is fundamental to health, and they teach techniques for slowing the breath or controlling the breath rate. The problem with that approach is that for most people, it is impossible to slow the breath without resorting to tension or overuse of accessory respiratory muscles. As a result, the long-term outcome is usually exacerbated hyperventilation, reliance on accessory respiratory muscles, and stress.

Still, learning how to allow the breath to *naturally* slow down can be beneficial. Often, we've become accustomed to breathing too rapidly, and therefore we do so simply out of habit rather than out of need.

Listening to the cues of the body and waiting for the gentle prompting for the next in-breath, we can re-familiarize ourselves with the natural, slower rhythms of normal breathing.

There are three phases to a normal, restful breath: inhalation, exhalation, and a pause at the bottom of the exhalation. As you have already learned, the inhalation is the only active portion of breathing. As such, this is the only portion of the breath that you can or should control in any way and therefore is the only portion that you can slow without stressing or abusing respiratory muscles.

There is no benefit to be had by excessively slowing the inhalation. However, if you consciously slow the inhalation just slightly, you can gain finer control and awareness of the movement. This will allow you to smooth the inhalation and focus the effort on the diaphragm. So, as part of a practice of slightly slowing the breath, experiment with gently slowing the inhalation so that it is smooth and controlled. A normal, healthy, smooth inhalation should last no longer than two to three seconds. It is a short, gentle, small movement that uses only the diaphragm. The chest should remain still and relaxed.

Next, the exhalation should be relaxed and completely effortless. Do not make any effort to control it. However, you may notice that by consciously relaxing the chest, abdomen, and the rest of the body deeply and completely, the exhalation will naturally be longer than the inhalation. Normal restful exhalations will likely last anywhere from four seconds upwards. Often the exhalation is either cut short or forced because of unnecessary muscular tension or effort.

Finally, at the bottom of the exhalation, a natural pause can occur. As with the exhalation, you should not do anything to force or extend a pause. Simply relax as deeply as possible to allow for a pause to occur naturally. Do not be concerned if a pause does not happen, but at the same time, be aware of the habit of inhaling before the onset of air hunger. As the exhalation completes, continue to relax deeply and wait for air hunger to appear before you start the cycle again with the next smooth, gentle inhalation.

Relax, Relax, Relax

The best thing you can do to improve your breathing is to relax! Breathing is an automatic function that requires no effort on your part. And, in most cases, disturbed breathing patterns will return to normal given enough time, if you simply relax, relax, relax.

The exercises I have suggested in the preceding two sections can be very helpful in re-training the breath to a normal pattern. That is because disturbed breathing patterns are often created by habits of hyperventilation and adaptation to hyperventilation. But these patterns are further reinforced through tension. So the more you relax and let go of any muscular tension, the more the body can naturally restore a normal breathing pattern.

Dangers of Breath Holds

For the most part, breath holds are harmful. That is because most breath holds are done unconsciously as part of conditioned habits. They interrupt normal, rhythmic breathing patterns, the result of which is inefficient breathing and the resultant compensatory measures in the body, which impair metabolism and all aspects of health.

Therefore, the best thing you can do regarding breath holds is to become aware of when you hold your breath and to relax and allow normal breathing to resume. We often develop the habit of holding our breath under stress or in times of fear, anxiety, or worry. These habits are self-defeating, and the more you can soften and allow normal breathing to resume, the better you will be for it.

Many breathing philosophies teach breath holds and claim that *consciously* holding the breath at certain times offers therapeutic benefits. While some forms of breath holding may be valuable, in most cases I believe it is not.

And in many cases, holding the breath can be unnecessarily harmful.

There are essentially three stages at which one can hold the breath: at the top of the inhalation, at the bottom of the exhalation, and during either the inhalation or exhalation.

Holding the breath at the top of the inhalation is the classic way most of us learn to hold our breath as children. It puts stress on the lungs and the structures of the lungs such as the bronchioles and alveoli, which can cause potential damage. If one is not hyperventilating, then the volume of air at the top of the inhalation will not be enough to do serious damage to the lungs. However, if one is hyper-inflating the lungs by hyperventilating, then the pressure is more likely to harm the lungs.

Holding the breath at the bottom of the exhalation offers the greatest therapeutic benefit, though the effects of this type of breath hold are not well studied. If one is forcefully exhaling beyond the point of expulsion of tidal volume, then this could place undue stress on the lungs to hold the breath in this state. But if one is not hyperventilating, then holding the breath at the bottom of the exhalation puts little stress on the lungs.

Holding the breath on inhalation or exhalation is unlikely to put a great deal of stress on the lungs, if one is not hyperventilating.

The primary benefit of conscious breath-holding is that it allows for a greater tolerance of carbon dioxide and possibly a greater tolerance of lower levels of oxygen. When breath holds are done correctly, the practice can produce results more quickly than simple reduced-breathing exercises. However, over time, breath holds don't offer any major benefits that cannot be obtained with simple reduced-breathing exercises.

Apart from the (small) risk of injury, the other drawback to breath holds is that you can train your body to form an unhealthy habit of holding your breath at the wrong times. Since a natural pause occurs at the bottom of the exhalation, this is the most sensible place to hold the breath if you are determined to do so. Holding your breath at other times can be detrimental because it will train you to hold your breath in unnatural parts of the breath cycle.

I don't wish to officially endorse breath holds. However, I realize that many people will practice them anyway. If you wish to practice breath holds, then I will offer a few suggestions for safe practice. To begin with, become proficient at breathing through the nose with reduced volume and while completely relaxed. That is a prerequisite for safe breath holding. Then, I suggest you do breath holds only at the bottom of the exhalation. Hold the breath for only so long as you can so that the next inhalation is normal, and the next exhalation is unforced and relaxed.

Any breath hold will be stressful. If you hold your breath minimize the stress by doing two things. First, hold the breath for short periods of time that you can incorporate into a regular pattern of breathing. So instead of holding the breath for long periods of time at irregular intervals, it is better to hold the breath for short periods of time that you can maintain across many breath cycles. This is sensible because regular, rhythmic patterns are preferred by the body.

Secondly, as you hold your breath, relax your body. By relaxing, you minimize the stress and train your body to accept the results more readily.

Emotions

S tressful and chaotic breathing patterns correlate with unpleasant emotional states such as anxiety and panic. This association has long been known, though various researchers and "experts" argue over whether there is any causative relationship between breathing and emotion. Still, anecdotally, many people find that calming the breath and restoring normal breathing patterns has beneficial effects on their emotional experiences.

Hyperventilation – as well as unhealthy breath holds – is common during times of stress. Start to notice how you are breathing (or not) during times of stress, and see what happens if you consciously calm the breath, relax the muscles, and allow for a normal breathing pattern to resume. Many people find that this has a very positive effect on their emotional state.

Unfortunately many people give the well-intended but bad advice to "take a deep breath" when feeling stressed. If you are in the habit of taking a deep breath (meaning a large breath in this case) then experiment with relaxing the tension of the chest and abdomen and allowing a normal breathing pattern to arise.

Because many of us have unconsciously developed a habit of relying on dysfunctional breathing patterns as strategies for dealing with stress, relaxing and allowing a normal breathing pattern can sometimes leave one feeling vulnerable in times of stress. If you find that this happens, then I suggest that you relax your muscles even more deeply. Allow an effortless, easy, relaxed normal breathing pattern to occur.

Dangerous Breathing Practices

There are many instructors, books, videos, and philosophies that teach extreme breathing practices without proper cautions, and I believe that this is dangerous. Of particular note are Holotropic Breathwork, Rebirthing Breathwork, and various forms of yogic pranayama.

Both Holotropic Breathwork and Rebirthing Breathwork are alternative therapies founded on the notion that many problems are the result of birth traumas. These therapies (and similar ones) utilize hyperventilation with the belief that it can offer some therapeutic benefits. (I am well aware that some instructors of these processes claim that they are not teaching hyperventilation. However, strictly speaking, the breathing patterns that they teach *will* most definitely produce hyperventilation in the overwhelming majority of people.)

I have done sessions of both of these types of therapies, and based on my experiences, the experiences of those around me, and my present understanding of breathing biology, I believe that these practices are unlikely to offer any long-term benefits, and in the short term they are potentially dangerous. They can and often do produce strong respiratory alkalosis, hypocalcemia, and a whole host of symptoms, including tetany – involuntary muscle contractions.

I also was a long-time student of yoga in various forms, including many classes in the hatha yoga style, as well as kundalini yoga. The instructors of these classes often guide students through various breathing exercises called pranayama or kriyas. Many of these exercises are unlikely to be particularly harmful, but at the same time they are unlikely to be particularly beneficial if they are done in the context of chronic poor breathing habits. But many of the exercises are potentially harmful.

Some examples of potentially harmful yogic breathing exercises include kapalbhati and bhastrika, because both of these exercises require extremely unnatural breathing patterns complete with forceful exhalations. Advocates of these pranayama claim that they are "energizing." However, most people are likely to experience a stress response. This may be mistaken for an "energized" feeling, but it is not healthy.

I do not wish to denigrate yogic breathing practices as a whole. Some gentle exercises have been shown to have potentially beneficial effects. For example, alternate nostril breathing can have positive effects. However, many are potentially dangerous, especially when practiced without expert guidance. I am perfectly happy to concede that there is a possibility that some of the extreme pranayama may offer benefits in the right context. But my understanding of human biology doesn't suggest any reason to believe that they offer any benefits to most people most of the time. And most of us will be far better off not practicing them. We can gain the most benefit from relaxing into a normal breathing pattern.

Devices

There are various devices that are sold as breathing training aids. Many focus on resisting inhalation. I believe that these devices are unlikely to be very helpful in restoring a normal breathing pattern. It is possible that they can offer benefits to some people, but I think there are better options. And, in fact, if one uses these devices with the intention of breathing more deeply (which is how the devices are sometimes marketed), then they may be counterproductive, if one wishes to restore healthy breathing.

The only device that I have come across that I like is the Frolov device, or the U.S. knock-off (for half the price) called BreathSlim. This device uses water to provide resistance for either the inhalation or the exhalation or both. And I find that resistance on exhalation is often far more beneficial than resistance on the inhalation. That is because the gentle resistance on exhalation trains the muscles in the chest and abdomen to relax.

I do not believe that any devices are necessary for the purpose of restoring normal breathing. However, I think that the Frolov or BreathSlim device can be a valuable aid for some people. I personally like using them.

The Frolov device comes with good instructions. However, the BreathSlim is half the price of the Frolov device. Yet the BreathSlim does *not* come with good instructions. So here, I will offer you some simple guidance on how to use either device.

When you use the device, you will be breathing at least partially through your mouth. In every other exercise, breathing through the mouth is a big no-no. However, it is essential for using the Frolov or BreathSlim device, and therefore it is okay for this purpose.

To begin with, fill the device with water below the recommended level. This will give less resistance and allow you to familiarize yourself with the exercises. As you become comfortable, you can increase the water level for more resistance.

First, inhale through the nose and exhale through the mouth. This will give no resistance on the inhalation and gentle resistance on the exhalation. For many people, it will require some days or weeks before graduating from this stage. You will know you are ready to move on when you are able to sustain a normal, reduced, and completely relaxed normal breathing cycle while exhaling through the device. The device requires that you reduce the breathing volume and have a gentle exhalation to prevent water from bubbling out of the device. So you will receive feedback from the device in this manner as you practice.

Once you are ready to move on to the next stage, you can begin to both inhale and exhale through the device. This stage is often considerably more challenging, because not only does the device provide resistance, it also increases the so-called dead space, meaning the area in which expelled air can reside without exiting the breathing system. That is because the device captures some of the exhaled air, which is then re-inhaled on the next breath. The result is that some of the inhaled air will contain a greater carbon dioxide content than you are accustomed to. This will increase the carbon dioxide content of the lungs.

If you find that inhaling and exhaling through the device is too difficult, then resist the impulse to increase the volume of your breath. You should be striving to reduce the volume of the breath to avoid hyperventilating. So instead, you can try several things.

First, try reducing the water level. If you already have a low water level and cannot reduce it more, then increase the water level and practice exhaling through the device while inhaling through the nose again. Then, when you become comfortable with that, reduce the water level and both inhale and exhale through the device.

Alternatively, you can try inhaling through the device and exhaling through the nose for a while to become comfortable with that. By doing so, you will be making it easier because you will not be increasing the dead space, meaning the concentration of carbon dioxide in the inhaled air will be normal.

Eventually, you will want to learn how to inhale and exhale through the device so that you can sustain a normal rhythm and reduced volume for four to five minutes at a time. Then, as you become comfortable, you can gradually increase the water level.

Unlike the simple reduced breathing exercise I shared with you earlier, I believe it is best not to practice with a Frolov or BreathSlim device too often. Once or twice a day for 10-20 minutes is plenty.

Again, I don't believe that it is necessary to use a device to restore a natural, normal breathing pattern. I strongly suggest that you practice breath awareness, diaphragmatic breathing, and simple reduced breathing before you consider getting a Frolov or BreathSlim device. These free methods can give you all the same benefits over time *and* they are a prerequisite for using the Frolov or BreathSlim device, even if you decide you want to use a device as a training aid. That is because you want to already have good breathing habits in place before you start with the device. Otherwise, using the device can be stressful and too difficult to obtain any benefits.

Compensation

It is worth noting that hyperventilation can be caused by habit or it can be a compensatory measure on the part of the body. There are many conditions that can lead to what is known as metabolic acidosis, which is a state in which the blood pH drops beyond the normal ability of the body to keep it within a narrow range. In order to compensate for metabolic acidosis, the body will resort to hyperventilation. As we've already seen throughout the book, hyperventilation reduces the blood concentration of carbon dioxide. That will normalize the pH of the blood, but it comes at a cost – as we've also seen – since hyperventilation produces a whole bunch of undesirable side effects.

Correcting hyperventilation is ultimately going to be helpful since it was only masking an underlying imbalance. But to do so, you'll probably need to address the underlying problem, as well. The underlying causes of metabolic acidosis are many, but some of them include renal failure, chronic renal failure, and intoxication from various drugs and chemicals.

In the case of intoxication, particularly if chronic, then it is a good idea to remove the intoxicants. Some of the intoxicants that can cause metabolic acidosis are chemicals that one may be exposed to through occupation. For example, ethanol, methanol, formaldehyde, ethylene glycol, and toluene are all possible causes. Drugs such as metformin, bile acid sequestrants, salicylates (such as aspirin or in some herbs, such as willow or meadowsweet), and acetazolamide all can produce metabolic acidosis, as well. And, as already mentioned, ethanol, which is found in large quantities in alcoholic beverages (it *is* the alcohol in alcoholic beverages) can produce metabolic acidosis. So for anyone experiencing metabolic acidosis, it would be best to avoid or reduce exposure to these substances.

In cases of renal failure or chronic renal failure, some studies have demonstrated that increasing alkaline minerals in the body can help. The most common substance used to assist in improving renal function is sodium bicarbonate (baking soda). A study published in the Journal of the American Society of Nephrology states that "bicarbonate supplementation slows the rate of progression of renal failure to [end stage renal disease] and improves nutritional status among patients with [chronic kidney disease]." That's a pretty conservative statement, but it does confirm that supplementation with baking soda may be helpful for those with renal failure.

Potassium citrate is another alkalizing supplement that is used in the medical community to help with acid conditions involving the kidneys. Specifically, potassium citrate is used to reduce symptoms and risk of uric acid kidney stones and gout, both of which are acidic conditions. And although I don't know of any human trials examining the effects of potassium citrate on renal function, there is at least one study published in the Journal of the American Society of Nephrology which concludes that the rats in the study given potassium citrate experienced significant improvement in kidney function.

Most studies and most people like to use strong supplements to achieve quick and dramatic results. And while it is possible to use both sodium bicarbonate and potassium citrate safely, a less heroic approach may be more appropriate for most people. Simply put, those experiencing metabolic acidosis *may* benefit from including more alkalizing foods in their diets. Typically, that means including more fruits and vegetables (including starchy vegetables such as potatoes, which are high in potassium). A study published in the American Journal of Clinical Nutrition found that an alkaline diet may help to reduce acidic state in the body. Although some breathing instructors recommend a raw, vegan diet (which would be very alkalizing), I believe that advice is misguided. Too much alkalinity is as much a problem as too much acidity. Furthermore, those extreme diets tend to create other metabolic problems, most notably decreased metabolic rate. As I have written about extensively in other books, eating enough and a variety of foods is very important for health. Please do not be misled. Simply be sure to include adequate fruits and vegetables in your diet, in addition to everything else that you eat.

Finally, magnesium deficiencies can contribute to acidic states, leading to hyperventilation. Unfortunately, hyperventilation also leads to increased magnesium excretion, which is a vicious cycle. Reportedly, for many people supplemental magnesium can be helpful initially. As the breath normalizes, the need for supplemental magnesium will decrease, since the body won't be excreting so much. Most people find that chelated magnesium as magnesium citrate, malate, or glycinate is best tolerated. Do not take too much because excess magnesium will cause gastrointestinal upset and a laxative effect. Some people also report that soaking in Epsom salt (magnesium sulfate) baths is helpful as a way to absorb magnesium, and it may be better tolerated if oral supplementation is too laxative.

In conclusion, hyperventilation can sometimes be habitual, but other times it is compensatory. When it is compensatory, it is important and necessary to correct the underlying imbalance. There are some safe, natural ways that most people can explore how to correct the imbalance, including reducing exposure to problem drugs and chemicals. Also, for some people, increasing fruit and vegetable intake and supplementing with magnesium can be helpful. For people with diagnosed renal failure, you may want to speak with your doctor about the possible pros and cons of supplementing with baking soda or potassium citrate.

Parting Words

My sincere hope is that this book has given you a whole new view on breathing. And if you were to get only one thing from this book, I would want it to be this: relax deeply and trust in the body to breathe intelligently, perfectly, and normally as you let go ever more deeply in each moment.

Throughout the book, I have offered you insights into the anatomy and biology of breathing. Of course, this is meant only to demonstrate that there is good evidence to support the notion that relaxed, easy, gentle, natural breathing is best. None of what I have written is intended to say that there is only ever one right way to breathe for all people and in all circumstances. There are lots of factors to keep in mind. But when you understand how the body breathes, why it breathes, and what the requirements are, you are in a better position to relax and let go, to breathe *easily* instead of deeply.

The practices that I have offered you in this book are merely guidelines for you to explore and experiment. Based on everything I have learned and everything that I have experienced, I truly believe that the guidelines are safe, gentle, and promote good health. Give them a try. And do so *gently*. Remember that while restoring a normal breathing pattern may entail moments of slight discomfort, it should not be stressful nor should it *ever* cause pain. Always listen to your body's feedback, and be gentle with yourself. Remember that you have a lifetime to breathe!

Get My Future Books FREE

If you enjoyed this book (Hey, if you made it this far it couldn't have been that bad), you'll probably enjoy many of my other books about health and wellness. And you can get all my new releases in health and wellness for free by signing up for my mailing list at www.joeylotthealth.com. It's simple, it's free, and it's totally honest and legitimate. Nothing scammy or spammy or anything else like that (i.e. I won't be trying to sell you The 7 Dirty Underground Top Secret Weird Tricks for Rock Hard Abs or Young Living Oils). It's just about free books for those who appreciate my work, because I appreciate YOU. Simple as that.

Connect with Me

I welcome your questions, comments, and feedback of any kind. Please feel free to email me at joeylott@gmail.com. I am now receiving so many emails that I cannot always reply to each one, but I do read them all, and I do my best to reply to as many as possible. For the benefit of others, I may choose to publish my response to your email on my blog or in book format. I will maintain your privacy and anonymity, should I choose to publish my response.

One Small Favor

My sincere goal in writing is to share something that may be of value to you. And I endeavor to do so while keeping the costs low for readers. The success of my books and my ability to reach other readers who may benefit from my books depends in large part on having lots of thoughtful, honest reviews written about my work. You would do me a great favor if you would please take a moment to generously write a review of this book at Amazon.com. This will only take a few minutes of your time, and you will be helping me a great deal. I sure would appreciate it.

About the Author

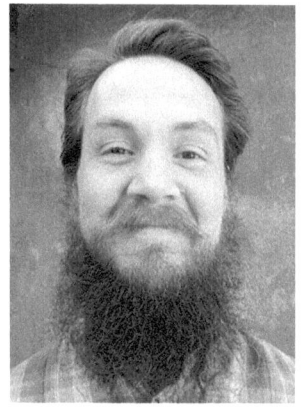

"The secret to happiness is to let go of everything - see through every assumption."

Beginning at a young age Joey Lott experienced intensifying anxiety. For several decades he lived with restrictive eating disorders, obsessions, compulsions, and an inescapable fear. By the time he was 30 years old he was physically sick, emotionally volatile, and mentally obsessed with keeping any and all unwanted thoughts and experiences at bay.

At this time Lott was living on a futon mattress in a tiny cabin in the woods. He was so sick that he could barely move. He was deeply depressed and hopeless. All this despite doing all the "right" things such as years of meditation, yoga, various "perfect" diets, clean air, and pure water.

Just when things were at their most dire, a crack appeared in the conceptual world that had formerly been mistaken for reality. By peering into this crack and underneath all the assumptions that had been unquestioned up to that moment, Lott began a great undoing. The revelation of this undoing is that reality is utterly simple, ever-present, seamless, and indivisible.

Lott's books provide a glimpse into the seamless, simple, and joyous nature of reality, offering a glimpse through the crack in conceptual worlds. Whether writing about the ultimate non-dual nature of reality, eating disorders, stress, disease, or any other subject, he offers the invitation to look at things differently, leaving behind the old, out-grown, painful limitations we have used to bind ourselves in suffering. And then, he welcomes you home to the effortless simplicity of yourself as you are.

Not sure where to begin? Pick up a copy of Lott's most popular book, *You're Trying Too Hard*, which strips away all the concepts that keep us searching for a greater, more spiritual, more peaceful life or self.

www.ingramcontent.com/pod-product-compliance
Lightning Source LLC
Chambersburg PA
CBHW050516290526
45786CB00007B/2590